C000121383

ACAP:

Augmentative Communication
Assessment Profile

ACAP:
Augmentative Communication Assessment Profile

Helena Goldman

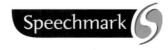

Speechmark Publishing Ltd
Telford Road, Bicester, Oxon OX26 4LQ, UK

Please note that in this text, for reasons of clarity alone, 'he' is used to refer to the child and 'she' to the practitioner.

If the enclosed acetate overlay is misplaced, a photocopiable master can be found in Appendix F. If this is used, any in-text references to yellow boxes on the overlay should be taken to refer to those with asterisks.

First published in 2002 by
Speechmark Publishing Ltd
Telford Road, Bicester, Oxon, OX26 4LQ, UK

www.speechmark.net

© Helena Goldman, 2002

All rights reserved. The whole of this work, including all text and illustrations, is protected by copyright. No part of it may be copied, altered, adapted or otherwise exploited in any way without express prior permission, unless it is in accordance with the provisions of the Copyright Designs and Patents Act 1988 or in order to photocopy or make duplicating masters of those pages so indicated, without alteration and including copyright notices, for the express purposes of instruction and examination. No parts of this work may otherwise be loaded, stored, manipulated, reproduced, or transmitted in any form or by any means, electronic or mechanical, including photocopying and recording, or by any information, storage and retrieval system without prior written permission from the publisher, on behalf of the copyright owner.

002-4766/Printed in the United Kingdom/1030

British Library Cataloguing in Publication Data

Goldman, Helena
   ACAP : augmentative communication assessment profile
   1. Handicapped – Means of communication   2. Autistic children
   I. Title
   618.9'28982

ISBN 0 86388 286 2

Contents

Acknowledgements

ACAP was the result of work covering a number of years, and particularly of working with children at Uffculme Primary Special School in Birmingham. I wish to thank all the children and the staff at the school. The children have taught me so much, but particularly that they are first and foremost individuals who happen to have something called autism.

I am also indebted to Mike Edwards for his patience in helping me to become computer literate.

Very special thanks are due to Helen Baldwin, Maggie Clifford, Lynne Conboy and Alex MacDonald for sharing their knowledge and skills, and especially for their sense of humour, encouragement and friendship.

Helena Goldman

The Augmentative Communication Assessment Profile (ACAP)

Background information

Professionals are continually challenged as to how to identify the communication system which will be of the most benefit to the non-verbal[1] child with an Autistic Spectrum Disorder (ASD). Picture- and object-trading systems, sign language and picture-pointing systems are common communication methods for this client group, but the choice of method taught to a child is largely dependent on the views, experience and policies of the child's speech and language therapist and/or teacher.

Practitioners who have a high level of experience with children on the autistic spectrum may have few difficulties in identifying the most beneficial alternative or augmentative communication (AAC) method. However, this decision is frequently based on personal experience and 'instinct' rather than on any objective assessment. This means that the chosen augmentative communication method may be implemented with a 'wait and see' attitude, as the ultimate success of the identified method is as yet largely unknown.

The Augmentative Communication Assessment Profile (ACAP) was initially an informal assessment tool used at Uffculme School in Birmingham. It was devised with the intention of removing the ad hoc element involved in the selection of a low-technology communication system considered most suited to the skills and needs of non-verbal children with autism, and has become an integral part of assessment procedure at this school. It was subjected to a number of minor modifications before resulting in this present version. It is designed for practitioners who welcome some objective guidance to assist them in identifying a primary method of communication on an individual basis. In addition, ACAP indirectly provides a basis for the practitioner for setting objectives and targets in order to develop the child's communication skills.

This is an assessment for signing and low-technology communication methods only. Unless there is an additional neurological or physical impairment that compounds the communication difficulties (eg, cerebral palsy or Duchenne muscular dystrophy), high-technology AACs are generally not considered for this client group. Integral to ASDs is an inherent difficulty in understanding about communication and social interaction which is unique to this client group. Learning about communication and why and how we interact with others would not be greatly aided by the use of high-technology AACs. The 'cause and effect' features of such aids may also serve as communication distracters, and could therefore hinder rather than promote communication.

Practitioners agree that unless the correct type of communication system is matched closely to the child's level of ability and need, there is little chance that the child will achieve functional communication. If pitched too high (eg, sign language for someone who lacks the requisite skills in the areas of motor function, imitation, social development, symbolic development, language and communication), the AAC will not be effective in reducing the non-verbal individual's frustration and anxiety. As ineffective communication frequently leads to a variety of challenging behaviours, this is another reason for early identification of the type of augmentative communication method best suited to the individual.

It is imperative that the child fully understands the chosen method of communication, and that he is taught this in functional and meaningful situations. When this is not the case, his frustration levels may increase if, for instance, he is required to imitate or produce what are to him meaningless actions prior to having his needs fulfilled.

When considering an alternative communication method, the less experienced practitioners within the field of autism may fail to take into account some seemingly insignificant and obscure communication-linked behaviour, and aspects of skills that are peculiar to autism. Also many have adopted a blanket policy on AAC systems which may be based on tradition alone, and which does not take into account the current abilities and requirements of the individual.

Although it is common knowledge that it is essential to tailor communication systems to the needs and skills of non-verbal individuals without autism, this is not always evident where people with autism are concerned. Specialists continue to advocate that it is worthwhile to attempt to teach signing (generally Makaton or Paget Gorman signed speech) to all non-verbal children on the autistic spectrum. In spite of some considerable effort, this has often proved as unattainable as speech (in the immediate sense) for this section of the population. Nevertheless, a small minority of the ASD population have become successful and competent users[2] of signed communication systems. While ACAP endeavours only to identify effective *expressive* means of communication for non-verbal individuals, the author readily acknowledges that in the *receptive* sense, standardised gesture and signs (particularly when having a strong descriptive component) can be of great value when used to support the giving of information and instructions.

In the last decade the use of picture-based trading communication systems has become very popular. These have been embraced to the extent that in some places they are used with all non-verbal children. As communication systems, they are generally more successful than sign language because they rely on the acquisition of very few skills. However, they are cumbersome for the more able child with a large requesting or commenting vocabulary. While picture-trading communication systems are very effective for people with a severe learning disability and autism, they have limitations where the more able child is concerned. By the very nature of the system, communication can become contrived and is subjected to restrictions similar to high-technology communication systems (eg, constraints of portability, rhythm and timing of interactions). For this group a more portable and less awkward system (eg, picture-pointing communication[3]) would be more effective in reducing anxiety and frustration.

Some practitioners have attempted laborious speech-production training over many hours, with virtually no functional result. Should the practitioner wish to persevere with speech-production training, it is advisable first to address the issue of functional communication. When the intervention emphasis is entirely on the aspect of speech production, it is wise for the practitioner to examine her reasons for this focus. Whatever the aims are, she needs to remember that speech must not be confused with communication, as an ability to speak does not mean that the person with autism automatically knows how to use this speech to communicate.

---

1 The term 'non-verbal' may include those who produce speech, but who may echo words and sentences and may even recite large chunks of favourite books or television jingles, yet are unable to use speech to communicate even the most basic of needs.

2 The expression 'successful and competent users' is used in the broadest sense in relation to the non-verbal child with autism. 'Successful and competent' implies that the child spontaneously and consistently signs legibly to communicate wants and needs.

3 The term 'picture-pointing communication' should more accurately be termed 'symbol-pointing communication', as this system may consist of more abstract symbols or written words. However, for the purpose of ACAP, the term 'picture-pointing' is more descriptive, as the majority of communicators using this method understand only a communication code which is more representational – eg, photographs and clear line drawings.

About the
Assessment Profile

Information gathered about the characteristics and skills of successful communicators using signing and the two main methods of low-technology communication (picture-based trading systems, and picture-pointing communication) formed the basis of ACAP. The information was collected over a number of years, while working with children with a wide variety of special needs associated with verbal communication impairment: for example, acquired head injury, cerebral palsy, Down's syndrome, Duchenne muscular dystrophy, severe learning disability and profound multiple learning disability but primarily with ASDs.

The data was collected separately for two groups: individuals with autism and those without autism. Fundamental to this exercise was the view that those skills identified as requisites to the various communication methods for the *non*-autism group could not automatically be assumed to be adequate requisites for those *with* autism. The reason for this is that there is an additional and intriguing difficulty specific to individuals with autism, which renders it essential to look beyond an impairment in verbal communication and related areas: for example, motor skills, language, cognitive and social development. The difficulty for people with autism lies mainly in their lack of understanding *about* communication, rather than in any physical inability to speak. A high proportion of these children can articulate speech sounds, sing and recite entire books verbatim and intelligibly. So, for the majority of this group, their difficulty is primarily an *inability to communicate* rather than an *inability to speak*. For the purpose of ACAP assessment, individuals come into the 'non-verbal' category if they are unable to use what speech they have to communicate at least simple requests to have basic needs filled. However, a relatively small number of non-verbal children with autism also have difficulties with the production and sequencing of speech sounds (dyspraxia). This client group may remain mute as a result of the very nature of autism, as individuals with ASD are not generally responsive to conventional therapy methods involving physical intervention, verbal instruction and imitation.

Comparison of the two sets of accumulated data made it possible to identify a group of common 'core skills', which were then evaluated for each method of AAC, irrespective of diagnosis. These 'core skills', or features, were also applicable to the group of non-verbal children on the autistic spectrum.

Next, a few additional essential criteria were included, which were exclusive to the autism group. When present, these would likely constitute severe obstacles to communication development (eg, a lack of understanding of shared attention, and pervasive active avoidance of eye contact). These two, when combined, make up the 'essential criteria' in the Assessment Profile.

Finally, a number of highly relevant, but not necessarily essential, criteria were identified and included in the Profile. The 'essential skills' are clearly marked in the section 'Clarification of Assessment Criteria'.

In time, while these 'essential skills' items remained intact, the Assessment Profile was subjected to a number of adaptations and modifications before resulting in the present format. A completed profile clearly identifies the method of communication which is likely to be the most effective. *The successful identification of the most appropriate communication method is measured by the ease with which the child adopts the new method; to what extent he uses it, and how effective it is in meeting his needs.* If an appropriate method is identified, the child demonstrates – usually within a few training sessions in functional and motivating situations – that he has understood the method (that is, the 'how' using signs, pointing or handing pictures to the conversation partners). It may take longer to get the idea of the 'what' – finding the right picture on the board or remembering the correct sign (see 'Communication Methods and Communication Codes', page 18).

ACAP is based on the premise that the three main augmentative communication systems are linked to developmental achievements in the areas of receptive language, pragmatics, social skills, cognition, semantic skills and symbolic understanding. Figure 1 shows the apparent progression of the AACs and their links with meaningful and functional speech development. Emergence of verbal communication for these individuals is unpredictable and follows a non-sequential developmental pattern, which is a feature of autism. Functional speech development may thus result from the successful implementation of any of the AACs.

When examining the essential criteria for each method of communication, it is apparent that these require different levels of skills. Picture-pointing communication is dependent on more advanced levels of attention, visual and symbolic skills than picture-trading systems, which require only a few basic behavioural responses. By contrast, an individual considered for signed communication will have achieved relatively advanced levels of symbolic development, fine motor imitation skills and social (and pragmatic) skills, as well as having developed some comprehension of spoken language and/or situations. It is not surprising, then, that any physically able child (without an ASD) who has reasonable cognitive ability with pre-verbal intentional communication skills would fill all criteria for signed communication if assessed by the Profile. The Assessment Profile

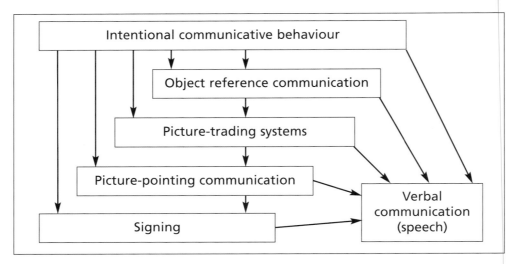

Figure 1: The progression of various AACs and their relationship with verbal communication

thus supports a view that the main AAC methods follow a sequence that is clearly linked to cognitive, social, language and skill development. Children with autism often learn skills out of the expected developmental sequence, and the same is true for the acquisition of alternative and augmentative communication methods (see Appendix E, page 41).

Who can administer ACAP?

ACAP can be administered by anybody who has a sound knowledge of communication and language as related to autism. Generally, this would include specialist speech and language therapists and specialist teachers.

Who does the Assessment cater for?

To date, the assessment has been used only with children on the autistic spectrum. Whilst ACAP covers some areas usually not considered when assessing other groups of non-verbal, physically able clients there is no reason why it would not be a helpful additional assessment tool for individuals with eg, Down's Syndrome.

What age-range does the Assessment cover?

Although so far ACAP has been used only with primary-school children (age-range of three to 11 years), it is thought to be appropriate for any age group.

What materials are required for completing the Assessment Profile?

No special materials are required, with the possible exception of Makaton (or other) symbols, and corresponding pictures for Assessment item 21.

An Overview of the Assessment Profile

It is essential to complete the pre-assessment section for each child before completing ACAP assessment. The child is not considered likely to comprehend one of the three more symbolic AACs, unless at the time of assessment affirmative answers are given to all of the following four questions:

- ◆ Does the child have at least fleeting attention skills?
- ◆ Have some intentional communicative behaviours been observed?
- ◆ Is there evidence that he can differentiate between people and objects?
- ◆ Does at least one item or activity motivate the child?

Until all of the above criteria have been achieved, work on intentional communication, joint attention skills, and/or object-reference communication is generally indicated.

The actual Assessment Profile consists of 27 closed questions, which directly or indirectly relate to communication (see Appendix A, page 25). These are in the following nine categories:

- ◆ Attention
- ◆ Visual skills
- ◆ Eye gaze
- ◆ Motor skills
- ◆ Physical proximity/touch
- ◆ Cognitive development
- ◆ Behaviour
- ◆ Receptive language development
- ◆ Communication status

Criteria as Identified for Each Method of Communication

Note: Essential criteria are indicated by an arrow and the numbers in parenthesis correspond to the behaviour criteria on the Assessment Profile form.

1 Criteria for any picture-trading communication system:

⟹ Fleeting attention skills

⟹ Differentiation between people and objects (5)

⟹ Motivation by at least one item/activity

⟹ Occasional, if fleeting, intentional communication

2 The potential picture-pointing communicator needs to exhibit a level of:

⟹ Visual scanning and discrimination skills (2)

⟹ Visual attention skills (1, 3)

⟹ Intentional communicative behaviours

⟹ Touch finger-pointing (16)

◆ Social awareness

◆ A degree of frustration when needs are not met

⟹ A concept of the representational/symbolic nature of pictures (23)

◆ Some verbal/situational understanding

3 The potential user of sign needs:

⟹ A high level of shared attention skills (1, 3)

◆ A degree of fine motor control

◆ Minimal or insignificant level of engagement in adopting alternating finger postures, hand-flapping or object-tapping

⟹ Intentional communicative behaviours (15)

⟹ A higher level of symbolic understanding (21), eg, recognising the Makaton/Rebus symbol for 'cat', and being able to match it to a more representative picture/photo of a cat

⟹ Reasonably accurate (recognisable) motor imitation ability (9)

◆ Some tolerance of physical proximity and prompts

◆ Social awareness

⟹ Basic communicative pointing skills (15)

◆ Imitation and understanding of social gesture

◆ No severe or profound autism or learning disability

Clarification of Assessment Criteria (ACAP)

CRITERION	CLARIFICATION
Attention	
❶ Can he sustain (one minute +) shared attention to an adult-directed activity?	The child has achieved Reynell's attention level 3 (attends to an adult-introduced activity, but this is entirely under the adult's control) for tasks that have a strong visual focus: eg, a simple book, lotto game.
Visual skills	
❷ Can he scan and complete a six-picture lotto board?	Visual scanning and matching skills (demonstrating concept of sameness).
❸ Can he attend to items to which an adult points in a simple picture?	The child understands that touch-pointing is an invitation/request to attend visually to the indicated item.
Eye gaze	
4 Does he consistently avoid looking at people?	The child consistently and actively avoids looking at others.
5 Does he differentiate between people and objects?	Does the child treat objects and people in the same way? Is it clear that he sees people as animate? Is there any indication of his viewing himself as belonging to this group?
Motor skills	
6 Does he have fine motor coordination difficulties?	Are the fine motor coordination difficulties so great that he cannot make reasonable approximations of the required hand shapes for Makaton or other signs?
7 Does he frequently engage in adopting unusual finger/hand postures, or hyper-extension of fingers?	If this is present, are the posturings so frequent as to be virtually constant unless required to hold objects (crayon, musical instrument, etc)?
8 Does he frequently arm-/hand-/finger-flap or tap items?	Is this type of behaviour virtually continuous?

Numbers in circles indicate communication board essential criterion.
Boxes with bold borders indicate sign-language essential criterion.

CRITERION	CLARIFICATION
9 Can he occasionally/consistently imitate a variety of one-hand gestures/movements: eg, waving, pointing?	Can he isolate right-hand movements from the left, or do bilateral symmetrical movements predominate? If imitations are only very occasional, do not answer 'yes' to this question.
10 Is he echopraxic?	This is the motor equivalent of echolalia. Answer 'yes' only if this is a consistent and virtually constant feature of the child's behaviour.
Physical proximity and touch	
11 Does he tolerate or accept physical prompts (occasionally/consistently)?	Does the child appear to experience considerable discomfort when close proximity and physical prompts are required?
12 Does he scratch/bite/pinch when physically prompted (consistently/frequently)?	Are these adverse behavioural responses a common response to physical prompting?
Communication status	
13 Does he eye-point to wanted items?	This is more than just looking at a wanted item. In order to answer 'yes', the child has to communicate the eye-point by then glancing at the adult to check if the message has been understood.
14 Does he take the adult to the desired object?	This is not using the adult's hand as a tool by 'throwing/pushing' it in the direction of the wanted item. Does the child see the *whole* person and not just the hand? Does he push or pull the adult (this need not be by holding the adult's hand) towards the object?
15 Does he gesture/distance finger-point to wanted object?	This is a gesture that must include communicative intent. Does the child gesture to the item, and then in some way check that this has been understood by the adult?
⑯ Can he touch-point?	This is not just the motor act of placing the finger (or thumb, or fist and thumb) on an item. Communicative intent has to be displayed in order to answer 'yes'.
Behaviour	
17 Is he aloof or passive?	Does the child remain uninvolved in his surroundings? Does he treat people as though inanimate?

Numbers in circles indicate communication board essential criterion.
Boxes with bold borders indicate sign-language essential criterion.

CRITERION	CLARIFICATION
18 Is he frustrated when wants/needs are not understood?	Does the child react if a need or want is not met?
19 Is he excessively noise-sensitive, and so frequently puts his fingers in his ears?	Would this behaviour prevent him from using sign-language effectively? This has to be a virtually constant behaviour in order to answer 'yes'.

Cognitive development

20 Does he have difficulties taking in information from more than one channel at a time?	Does the child encounter difficulties if information/instructions are presented visually as well as verbally? Does he do markedly better if only visual presentations are used for new or unfamiliar activities?
21 Can he match symbols to pictures?	Does he recognise stylised line drawings? Can he match these to colour pictures representing the same objects? (Some of the more representative Makaton or Rebus symbols can be used for this assessment: eg, cat, washing, sitting and biscuit symbols.
22 Is he diagnosed to have a severe to profound learning disability or a severe to profound ASD?	If the child has a severe or profound learning disability or ASD, he is less likely to become a competent signer, although he may learn to use a handful of signs to support his primary means of communication.
23 Does he understand that pictures are representative?	Does he show any indication of having understood that a picture stands for the real object? Can he match objects to pictures? If shown a photograph of a familiar person or object, does he then look for the actual item/person?

Receptive language skills

24 Does he understand single words in context?	Does he respond appropriately to single word instructions in their appropriate contexts, eg, 'shoes' when getting dressed.
25 Does he understand single words without situational cues?	Same as 24, but no obvious situational cues.
26 Does he demonstrate understanding of standard social gestures: eg, 'shhh', 'stop', 'come'?	Does he respond appropriately when these common gestures are used in their contexts?
27 Does he imitate standard social gestures: eg, 'shhh', 'bye-bye', etc?	Does he frequently imitate these social gestures in their appropriate contexts?

Numbers in circles indicate communication board essential criterion.
Boxes with bold borders indicate sign-language essential criterion.

Administration

The examiner should be well acquainted with the content of the Profile prior to the assessment. Please see the chart entitled 'Clarification of Assessment Criteria' on pages 10–12. It is recommended that focused observation methods are used to assess the child in a variety of naturally occurring contexts, with a view to collecting the required information to complete the Assessment Profile. Observation of the child in group teaching situations (such as the Literacy and Numeracy Hours, or story time), free play, snack time and singing would provide the examiner with the bulk of the required information. Additional information would include the views of parents and carers regarding the various alternative and augmentative communication methods, as well as any practical implications for their implementation in the home situation. This information is best sought via completion of the Pragmatics Profile of Early Communication Skills or another appropriate questionnaire focusing on the pragmatic aspects of language.

The actual completion of the Assessment Profile should take no longer than 15 minutes. The child need not be present, as the examiner should by then have available all relevant information as a result of her observations. The exception is item 21, which requires additional information. It is recommended that the child's speech and language therapist, teachers and the parents/carers in partnership consider the implications of the child's individual profile.

Procedure

1   Complete the pre-assessment section in Appendix A. page 25. Do not proceed with the assessment unless all pre-assessment criteria have been achieved.

2   Proceed to the second part of the form, and answer each question by referring to the section 'Clarification of Assessment Criteria'.

3   Should there be any uncertainty or disagreement regarding assessment criteria between the contributors to the assessment, mark these with a question mark in the relevant box.

4   When using the same form to review the individual's abilities, mark the shift in skills/development with an arrow to indicate direction of movement (see Appendix D, page 37). This information is thus

readily available should there be a need to trace communication progress at a later date. The assessment record form makes provision for re-assessment on a further three occasions.

Scoring

Do not include any inconclusive or inconsistent responses.

1   Count all white boxes containing an affirmative response, and record this score at the bottom of the form.

2   Repeat for the grey-tinted boxes.

3   If the majority of responses are recorded in white boxes, then look at the objectives marked in bold type on the form to ascertain if *all* five criteria have been met. If this is the case, proceed to 'Interpreting the results of ACAP'. If not, go to number 5 below.

4   If the majority of grey-tinted boxes are indicated, proceed to 'Interpreting the results of ACAP'.

5   If the responses fall fairly equally in both grey and white boxes, use the transparent overlay by placing it on the completed form, ensuring a careful match of the two. Ensure that all the yellow-coloured boxes are ticked. If this is the case, proceed to 'Interpreting the results of ACAP'.

Interpreting the results of ACAP

When completed, the record form becomes a visual profile of the child's alternative and augmentative communication skills and requirements. The pattern of ticked boxes, whether grey or white (or if the overlay is used, ticks in yellow boxes) gives an instant suggestion as to the child's best communication options at the time of assessment. However, further analysis of the results is necessary to ascertain that the identification of a communication method is accurate.

◆   In the event that the Profile shows that all five bold-type criteria have been filled, this would indicate that some form of signed communication is the method likely to most benefit the child (see Appendix B, page 39).

◆   If predominantly grey-tinted boxes are ticked, a picture-trading communication system such as the Picture for Object Trading

(POT)[1], or the Picture Exchange Communication System (PECS)[2] is indicated (see Appendix C, page 33).

◆ Analysis of a Profile frequently indicates that signing or picture-trading is not considered an effective communication option (see Appendix D, page 37). Use of the transparent overlay would suggest whether the child could be taught successfully some form of picture-pointing communication. All highlighted essential criteria (indicated by yellow colouring) must be ticked before considering implementing this form of communication. If not all yellow boxes are ticked, this shows that the individual would most readily learn effective communication by using a picture-trading system.

◆ Occasionally a child may present an erratic profile, which at first glance appears to indicate that he is unsuited to any of the AACs (see Appendix E, page 41). Further examination of this profile will show that this child has not achieved all the requisite skills for either signing or picture-pointing communication. Although the profile appears to suggest that picture-trading is not the best option, it is in fact the only functional option at the moment. The profile reveals that this child's level of skill is indicative of his moving away from this mode of AAC, and that this may soon prove inadequate in filling his communication needs. In the meantime, the profile provides the practitioner with valuable information concerning the identification of communication objectives for future intervention.

1 Picture for Object Trading (POT) was developed by Goldman,1998.
2 The author recognises that the developers of PECS do not necessarily agree with these requisite criteria.

Issues Relating to Assessment Findings

Quantitative approaches to analysis will not alone identify the method of alternative or augmentative communication most likely to benefit the individual. To illustrate this point, see Appendix D, page 37, where the number of pro-signing responses amounts to 18, while the pro-pointing communication responses number only 15. On examining the individual responses it is apparent that this child has not filled all essential pro-signing criteria (item 21), and signing at this stage is, therefore, not a functional option.

There may be instances when a child has filled all the criteria for one method of communication, but some of these responses were considered unreliable or tenuous. In this case it would be wise to opt for the communication method which has received the highest score, and for which all essential criteria have been met.

Some of the more able children successfully favour a combination of sign, picture-based communication method and speech, while showing a clear preference for one particular method. For instance, most picture-pointing communicators learn a small number of signs to complement their picture-based system. These signs generally refer to more abstract concepts which are difficult to depict, but which are fundamental to the development of independence skills: eg, 'help', 'more', 'stop', 'finished'. Likewise, users of sign often switch to using picture-pointing communication for certain concepts, or use this as a backup system for non-signing communication partners. It is not uncommon for some signing children to use sign competently in one context (eg, school), while preferring to use picture-pointing communication at home or in a respite setting. If the child is equally at ease with a combination of AACs, this is referred to as 'mixed AAC'.

Although it is always advisable to take the cues regarding methods of communication from the child and build on these, it is crucial to consider the practicality of the indicated method as related to the various contexts. The AAC method as indicated by the Profile always needs to be considered in relation to other information available about the child (eg, parents'/carers' views) before making a decision for or against any method. The child's primary means of communication should be decided only in consultation with his speech and language therapist, teacher, parents and carers. For instance, a signing system may not be feasible in a respite setting if carers are not comfortable with, or skilled in, this method of communication.

Communication Methods and Communication Codes

Equal in importance to the identification of a communication method is the selection of an appropriate communication code (ie, the type of signs or symbols used). Unless there is a careful match between an individual's level of development in the relevant areas and the selected symbol or sign system, the appropriate method alone will not ensure effective communication.

The skills of a specialist speech and language therapist are helpful but not essential for completing an ACAP assessment. However, it is strongly recommended that their input is sought for this stage. Information is needed on vocabulary selection, receptive language skills, social and pragmatic needs and competence, as well as an estimate of the individual's levels of semantic and symbolic understanding.

Sign systems

In the case of signed communication, the decision as to which system to use needs careful consideration. A common choice is Makaton signing, but many use Paget Gorman Sign System, or sometimes a careful marriage of the two. Makaton signing alone is not likely to cater for all the vocabulary needs of a person with autism.

Although the signing vocabulary of Makaton covers a wide range of functional concepts, it was not designed for people with autism. It has already been established that the chosen AAC system has to be functional and meet the communication needs of the individual. It follows, then, that this has to include his special interests and obsessions: eg, a wide variety of different types of trains, or obscure exotic animals. Signs from a wider system (eg, British Sign Language) may be incorporated for this needed additional information. It is wise to ensure that access to special interest vocabulary will be readily available for future needs.

When selecting individual signs, bear in mind the difficulty that people with autism have with abstractions and generalisations. If signs are too abstract, they are more difficult to learn than if an element of natural descriptive gesture is included. Beware of signs that are too specific and assume an understanding of semantic links. One very able person with autism, relates that, with her very literal level of processing, for instance, a milking motion to denote the concept of milk always leads her to think of the action of milking cows, and not milk.

Symbols

The code used to transmit the communication of needs and wants in picture-trading systems and picture-pointing communication must reflect the individual's level of symbolic and semantic knowledge. Are exact photographs of the items essential, for example, or will line-drawings like PCS Boardmaker icons suffice? Has the individual an understanding of black and white symbols like those of Makaton? If this is the case, it is important to check whether the child can generalise the symbol: eg, a stylised drawing of a glass meaning drink. Is it understood as one particular type of drink, eg, orange juice, or can it also stand for water or milk? Further assessment to ascertain whether the individual has categorisation skills is also useful. Can the same black glass outline stand as a symbol for a variety of drinks, irrespective of receptacle in which they are served: eg, hot tea in a cup, packet drinks with straws, fast-food milkshakes in paper cups, bottled water, etc. This would assist the practitioner who is designing the communication board, and ultimately would have a bearing on how successful the individual will be in using the selected method of communication.

Any alternative or augmentative method of communication requires a high level of commitment from all involved with the child's primary care. Prior to implementation, careful planning and vocabulary selection is vital for the system to become truly the child's primary communication system. Initial signs, symbols or pictures must be tailored to the child's individual special needs, interests and obsessions, as motivation to communicate is a prerequisite to any act of communication. Follow-up and continuation in the child's home (and respite care) environment is advisable to ensure effective communication. Generalisation of the indicated method may not be automatic, and the parents/carers need to be prepared to re-teach the communication system in the home and respite settings. If the child uses photographs or symbols, these would be likely to differ from those used at school, and consequently would need to be introduced in the same way as any new photographs or symbols.

The Pilot Study
and Findings

As mentioned previously, the Assessment Profile was initially an assessment that had been in use for a few years at Uffculme School in Birmingham. This is an early years and primary school for children with autism and severe communication disorders. The school accepts children from Birmingham and neighbouring areas, and the pupils represent a wide socio-economic and cultural mix. A few of the children in the study had had limited exposure to English prior to their admittance to the school.

External interest in the Profile necessitated the publication of existing data regarding validity in identifying the most functional method of communication. The completed Profiles to date were therefore collated and analysed, and formed the basis of this retrospective pilot study.

All non-verbal children with autism at the school during the school year 1998–9 were assessed on ACAP. These 31 children ranged in age from three to 11 years.

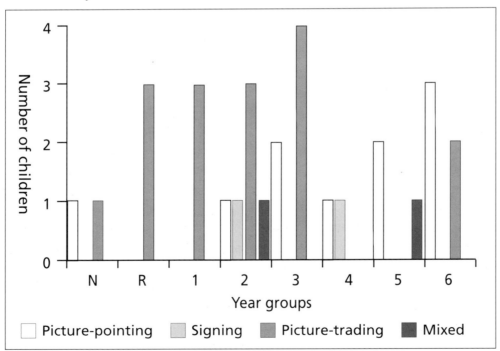

Figure 2: Distribution of identified methods of augmentative communication over year groups

The Assessment Profile proved valid for all 31 children, in that it accurately identified the method that best corresponded to the individuals' levels of skill and need. In the 11 cases where children were already using one of the three systems, there was concern that the Profile assessment could be subject to administration bias. Practitioners might be unintentionally inclined to err on the side of the communication method that the child was already using in an eagerness to show that their non-ACAP assessment of the child's AAC requirements was correct. To prevent this bias, these 11 profiles were each completed 'blind' by at least two members of staff.

Table 1: *Communication development of the children in the pilot study*

No speech sounds or words ('mute') – no means of communicating		Immediate echolalia – no communicative intent		Echolalia – communicative intent		Using an AAC method – no speech		Using combination of AACs and oral communication		Oral communication only	
Before	After	Before	After	Before	After	Before	After	Before	After	Before	After
11	0	5	0	4	0	6	1	5	14	0	4

Note: 'Before' refers to before ACAP assessment.
    'After' refers to the end of the school year. For some of the pupils this would mean a lapse of 10 months, but as children were admitted to the school throughout the year this was a variable period of time. In the case of one child, this meant a period of only six weeks.

In the early stages of the development of ACAP, it was incorrectly assumed that all children partaking in the assessment were capable of at least picture-trading communication. At this time the pre-assessment criteria were not yet identified, but when they were formally incorporated into the Profile it became apparent that four of the 31 children would not have met these criteria. These children, not surprisingly, encountered great difficulties in learning to trade pictures for objects. Communication progress of these four was slow, but after several months all of them had learnt to use photographs to communicate the preference for food and one or two favourite items (eg, a book or an electronic keyboard). Two years later they had mostly satisfied the pre-assessment criteria, but continue to have difficulties with the initiating aspect of communication, and will only make requests in response to verbal and gestural prompts. All four are diagnosed with severe to profound learning difficulties, and have severe to profound autism. Although, in the end, the children learnt to communicate basic needs to some extent, much time was spent in the actual teaching of the communication system. In retrospect, this time could have been better allocated to the teaching of intentionality and shared attention skills, as well as to the further development of the children's object-reference communication.

One child identified as a potential user of picture-pointing communication was the only one not using his identified means of AAC at the end of the school year. The parents were not in agreement with their child being taught an augmentative communication method.

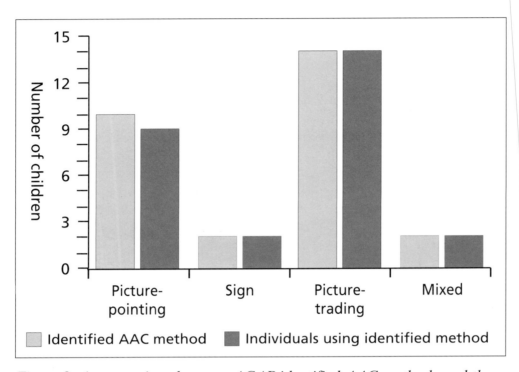

Figure 3: A comparison between ACAP-identified AAC methods and the number of children using this as a primary method of AAC at the end of the school year

Conclusion

ACAP has proved invaluable in assisting staff at Uffculme School to identify effective methods of communication for its non-verbal population. An added bonus of the assessment is that it highlights deficits in areas related to communication which can then be addressed directly by means of specific targets and objectives as part of the child's Individual Education Plan.

Therefore the Assessment Profile has proved to have a threefold value:

◆ It assists all involved in the decision concerning the most effective method of augmentative communication on an individual basis.
◆ It provides an objective overview of the individual's skills, which are requisite to communication.
◆ It charts progress of these skills as the child matures and develops.

Regular reassessment on the Profile is recommended, because experience has shown that as children mature and change, so do their communication skills and requirements. See Table 1, page 24 ('Communication development of children in the pilot study') and Appendix D, page 37, where the arrows indicate communication progress over a 10-month period.

Some individuals progress from a picture-based trading system directly to some level of oral communication. The majority of these children then use a picture-pointing communication system to augment their spoken language (which by then will have become their primary means of communication). This system may be necessary for some time, as it provides the individual with a degree of security. This is particularly true when the child is in new situations with less familiar adults, or in times of distress. If he is anxious, the new communication skill may be temporarily inaccessible, and a picture-based system may then be less demanding and therefore a useful tool to alleviate this stress. For this reason, it is strongly advised that the alternative method of communication be available even when the child has developed some functional spoken language.

Speech is always the ultimate goal for all children with autism, but for some it will prove unattainable. However, by consistently using an alternative communication system tailored to the child's special requirements and level of skills, he will develop at least a basic understanding of the act of communication. Only then can the repertoire of language functions be extended successfully (ie, progressing beyond requests to meet needs and wants). After a while, it is not unusual for some children (particularly those who have displayed immediate and delayed echolalia in the past) to start using these very words, or word approximations, spontaneously in their appropriate contexts, before developing further verbal communication skills.

ACAP gives practitioners objective guidance in their search for effective AAC methods based on information about the individual. At times, practitioners and parents may have a difference of opinion as to what constitutes the most appropriate type of alternative communication method. While it would be inadvisable to dissuade anybody from using a particular AAC solely on the basis of this assessment, ACAP can suggest the most effective method available at any given time in the child's development. It is, above all, in the child's interest to seek to identify a communication method that could quickly become an effective communication tool, and thus prevent the inevitable frustration that would result from the attempted teaching of what may, at the moment, be an inaccessible form of communication.

The Augmentative Communication Assessment Profile (ACAP)

ACAP

Client's name		DoB	
Date	Review Date	Review Date	Review Date
Profile completed by			

Present mode of communication

Indicated method of communication	**Date**
Object reference	
Picture-trading	
Picture-pointing	
Sign language	

Comments

PRE-ASSESSMENT CRITERIA

CRITERIA	YES	NO
◆ Has the client at least fleeting attention skills?		
◆ Have some intentional communicative behaviours been observed?		
◆ Is there evidence that he can differentiate between people and objects?		
◆ Is he motivated by at least one item/activity?		

Proceed with the assessment only if all four questions receive a 'yes' answer.

© Helena Goldman, 2002. This form may be copied for instructional use only.

ACAP

BEHAVIOUR	YES	NO
ATTENTION		
❶ **Can he sustain (1 minute+) shared attention skills to an adult-directed activity?**	☐	
VISUAL SKILLS		
❷ Can he scan and complete a six-picture lotto board?		
❸ **Can he attend to items that adult points to in a simple picture?**	☐	
EYE GAZE		
4 Does he consistently avoid looking at people?		
5 Does he differentiate between people and objects?		
MOTOR SKILLS		
6 Does he have fine motor coordination difficulties?		
7 Does he frequently engage in adopting unusual finger/hand postures or hyper-extension of fingers?		
8 Does he frequently arm/hand/finger flap or tap items?		
9 **Can he occasionally/consistently imitate a variety of one-hand gestures/movements, eg, waving, pointing?**	☐	
10 Is he echopraxic?		
PHYSICAL PROXIMITY/TOUCH		
11 Does he tolerate/accept physical prompts (occasionally/consistently)?		
12 Does he scratch/bite/pinch when physically prompted (consistently/frequently)?		
COMMUNICATION STATUS		
13 Does he eye point to wanted items?		
14 Does he take adult to object?		
15 **Does he gesture/distance finger-point to wanted object?**	☐	
⓰ Can he touch point?		
BEHAVIOUR		
17 Is he aloof/passive?		
18 Is he frustrated when (wants/needs) are not understood?		
19 Is he excessively noise-sensitive, and so frequently puts fingers in his ears?		
COGNITIVE BEHAVIOUR		
20 Does he have difficulties taking in information from more than one channel at a time?		
21 **Can he match symbols to pictures?**	☐	
22 Is he diagnosed as having a severe/profound learning disability /ASD?		
㉓ Does he understand that pictures are representative?		
RECEPTIVE LANGUAGE SKILLS		
24 Does he understand single words in context?		
25 Does he understand single words – no situational cues?		
26 Does he demonstrate understanding of standard social gestures, eg, 'shhh', 'stop', 'come'?		
27 Does he imitate standard social gestures, eg, 'shhh', 'bye-bye'?		

Suggested Primary Method of Communication

Signing = ___/27   Picture-trading = ___/27   Picture-pointing = ___/21

27

P © Helena Goldman, 2002. This form may be copied for instructional use only.

The Augmentative Communication Assessment Profile (ACAP)

Example of a Sign Language Profile

ACAP

BEHAVIOUR	YES	NO
ATTENTION		
❶ Can he sustain (1 minute+) shared attention skills to an adult-directed activity?	✔	
VISUAL SKILLS		
❷ Can he scan and complete a six-picture lotto board?	✔	
❸ Can he attend to items that adult points to in a simple picture?	✔	
EYE GAZE		
4 Does he consistently avoid looking at people?	✔	
5 Does he differentiate between people and objects?	✔	
MOTOR SKILLS		
6 Does he have fine motor coordination difficulties?		✔
7 Does he frequently engage in adopting unusual finger/hand postures or hyper-extension of fingers?		✔
8 Does he frequently arm/hand/finger flap or tap items?		✔
9 Can he occasionally/consistently imitate a variety of one-hand gestures/movements, eg, waving, pointing?	✔	
10 Is he echopraxic?		✔
PHYSICAL PROXIMITY/TOUCH		
11 Does he tolerate/accept physical prompts (occasionally/consistently)?	✔	
12 Does he scratch/bite/pinch when physically prompted (consistently/frequently)?		✔
COMMUNICATION STATUS		
13 Does he eye point to wanted items?	?	
14 Does he take adult to object?	✔	
15 Does he gesture/distance finger-point to wanted object?	✔	
❶❻ Can he touch point?	✔	
BEHAVIOUR		
17 Is he aloof/passive?		✔
18 Is he frustrated when (wants/needs) are not understood?		✔
19 Is he excessively noise-sensitive, and so frequently puts fingers in his ears?		✔
COGNITIVE BEHAVIOUR		
20 Does he have difficulties taking in information from more than one channel at a time?		?
21 Can he match symbols to pictures?		
22 Is he diagnosed as having a severe/profound learning disability /ASD?		✔
❷❸ Does he understand that pictures are representative?	✔	
RECEPTIVE LANGUAGE SKILLS		
24 Does he understand single words in context?	✔	
25 Does he understand single words – no situational cues?	✔	
26 Does he demonstrate understanding of standard social gestures, eg, 'shhh', 'stop', 'come'?	✔	
27 Does he imitate standard social gestures, eg, 'shhh', 'bye-bye'?	✔	

Suggested Primary Method of Communication

Signing = **23/27**   Picture-trading = 2/27   Picture-pointing = 16/21

© Helena Goldman, 2002. This form may be copied for instructional use only.

The Augmentative Communication Assessment Profile (ACAP)

Example of a Picture-trading Communication Profile

ACAP

BEHAVIOUR	YES	NO
ATTENTION		
❶ Can he sustain (1 minute+) shared attention skills to an adult-directed activity?	☐	?
VISUAL SKILLS		
❷ Can he scan and complete a six-picture lotto board?		?
❸ Can he attend to items that adult points to in a simple picture?	☐	?
EYE GAZE		
4 Does he consistently avoid looking at people?		✔
5 Does he differentiate between people and objects?		?
MOTOR SKILLS		
6 Does he have fine motor coordination difficulties?	✔	
7 Does he frequently engage in adopting unusual finger/hand postures or hyper-extension of fingers?	✔	
8 Does he frequently arm/hand/finger flap or tap items?	✔	
9 Can he occasionally/consistently imitate a variety of one-hand gestures/movements, eg, waving, pointing?	☐	✔
10 Is he echopraxic?		✔
PHYSICAL PROXIMITY/TOUCH		
11 Does he tolerate/accept physical prompts (occasionally/consistently)?	✔	
12 Does he scratch/bite/pinch when physically prompted (consistently/frequently)?	✔	
COMMUNICATION STATUS		
13 Does he eye point to wanted items?		✔
14 Does he take adult to object?		✔
15 Does he gesture/distance finger-point to wanted object?	☐	✔
⓰ Can he touch point?		✔
BEHAVIOUR		
17 Is he aloof/passive?	✔	
18 Is he frustrated when (wants/needs) are not understood?		✔
19 Is he excessively noise-sensitive, and so frequently puts fingers in his ears?	✔	
COGNITIVE BEHAVIOUR		
20 Does he have difficulties taking in information from more than one channel at a time?	✔	
21 Can he match symbols to pictures?	☐	✔
22 Is he diagnosed as having a severe/profound learning disability /ASD?	✔	
㉓ Does he understand that pictures are representative?		?
RECEPTIVE LANGUAGE SKILLS		
24 Does he understand single words in context?		?
25 Does he understand single words – no situational cues?		?
26 Does he demonstrate understanding of standard social gestures, eg, 'shhh', 'stop', 'come'?		✔
27 Does he imitate standard social gestures, eg, 'shhh', 'bye-bye'?		✔

Suggested Primary Method of Communication

Signing = 3/27   Picture-trading = **17/27**   Picture-pointing = 3/21

© Helena Goldman, 2002. This form may be copied for instructional use only.

The Augmentative Communication Assessment Profile (ACAP)

Example of a Picture-pointing Communication Profile

ACAP

BEHAVIOUR	YES	NO
ATTENTION		
❶ Can he sustain (1 minute+) shared attention skills to an adult-directed activity?	✔	
VISUAL SKILLS		
❷ Can he scan and complete a six-picture lotto board?	✔	
❸ Can he attend to items that adult points to in a simple picture?	✔	
EYE GAZE		
4 Does he consistently avoid looking at people?	✔	
5 Does he differentiate between people and objects?	✔	
MOTOR SKILLS		
6 Does he have fine motor coordination difficulties?		✔
7 Does he frequently engage in adopting unusual finger/hand postures or hyper-extension of fingers?	✔	
8 Does he frequently arm/hand/finger flap or tap items?	✔	
9 Can he occasionally/consistently imitate a variety of one-hand gestures/movements, eg, waving, pointing?	✔ ← ✔	
10 Is he echopraxic?		✔
PHYSICAL PROXIMITY/TOUCH		
11 Does he tolerate/accept physical prompts (occasionally/consistently)?	✔ ← ✔	
12 Does he scratch/bite/pinch when physically prompted (consistently/frequently)?		✔
COMMUNICATION STATUS		
13 Does he eye point to wanted items?	✔	
14 Does he take adult to object?	✔ ← ?	
15 Does he gesture/distance finger-point to wanted object?	✔ ← ?	
❶❻ Can he touch point?	✔ ← ?	
BEHAVIOUR		
17 Is he aloof/passive?	✔	
18 Is he frustrated when (wants/needs) are not understood?	✔	
19 Is he excessively noise-sensitive, and so frequently puts fingers in his ears?	✔	
COGNITIVE BEHAVIOUR		
20 Does he have difficulties taking in information from more than one channel at a time?	✔	
21 Can he match symbols to pictures?		✔
22 Is he diagnosed as having a severe/profound learning disability /ASD?		✔
㉓ Does he understand that pictures are representative?	✔	
RECEPTIVE LANGUAGE SKILLS		
24 Does he understand single words in context?	✔	
25 Does he understand single words – no situational cues?	✔	
26 Does he demonstrate understanding of standard social gestures, eg, 'shhh', 'stop', 'come'?	?	
27 Does he imitate standard social gestures, eg, 'shhh', 'bye-bye'?		✔

Suggested Primary Method of Communication

Signing = 18/27   Picture-trading = 8/27   Picture-pointing = **15/21**

P © Helena Goldman, 2002. This form may be copied for instructional use only.

The Augmentative Communication Assessment Profile (ACAP)

Example of an Atypical Picture-trading Communication Profile

ACAP

BEHAVIOUR	YES	NO
ATTENTION		
❶ Can he sustain (1 minute+) shared attention skills to an adult-directed activity?	✔	
VISUAL SKILLS		
❷ Can he scan and complete a six-picture lotto board?		✔
❸ **Can he attend to items that adult points to in a simple picture?**	✔	
EYE GAZE		
4 Does he consistently avoid looking at people?		✔
5 Does he differentiate between people and objects?	✔	
MOTOR SKILLS		
6 Does he have fine motor coordination difficulties?	✔	
7 Does he frequently engage in adopting unusual finger/hand postures or hyper-extension of fingers?	✔	
8 Does he frequently arm/hand/finger flap or tap items?		✔
9 **Can he occasionally/consistently imitate a variety of one-hand gestures/movements, eg, waving, pointing?**	✔	
10 Is he echopraxic?		✔
PHYSICAL PROXIMITY/TOUCH		
11 Does he tolerate/accept physical prompts (occasionally/consistently)?	✔	
12 Does he scratch/bite/pinch when physically prompted (consistently/frequently)?		✔
COMMUNICATION STATUS		
13 Does he eye point to wanted items?	✔	
14 Does he take adult to object?	✔	
15 **Does he gesture/distance finger-point to wanted object?**	✔	
❶❻ Can he touch point?	✔	
BEHAVIOUR		
17 Is he aloof/passive?		✔
18 Is he frustrated when (wants/needs) are not understood?	✔	
19 Is he excessively noise-sensitive, and so frequently puts fingers in his ears?		✔
COGNITIVE BEHAVIOUR		
20 Does he have difficulties taking in information from more than one channel at a time?	✔	
21 **Can he match symbols to pictures?**		✔
22 Is he diagnosed as having a severe/profound learning disability /ASD?	✔	
❷❸ Does he understand that pictures are representative?	?	
RECEPTIVE LANGUAGE SKILLS		
24 Does he understand single words in context?	✔	
25 Does he understand single words – no situational cues?		?
26 Does he demonstrate understanding of standard social gestures, eg, 'shhh', 'stop', 'come'?		✔
27 Does he imitate standard social gestures, eg, 'shhh', 'bye-bye'?	?	

Suggested Primary Method of Communication

Signing = 17/27   Picture-trading = **8/27**   Picture-pointing = 14/21

© Helena Goldman, 2002. This form may be copied for instructional use only.

The Augmentative Communication Assessment Profile (ACAP)

ACAP overlay to determine whether the client has met the criteria for picture-pointing communication

ACAP

BEHAVIOUR	YES	NO
ATTENTION		
❶	*	
VISUAL SKILLS		
❷	*	
❸	*	
EYE GAZE		
4		
5		
MOTOR SKILLS		
6		
7		
8		
9		
10		
PHYSICAL PROXIMITY/TOUCH		
11		
12		
COMMUNICATION STATUS		
13		
14		
15		
❶❻	*	
BEHAVIOUR		
17		
18		
19		
COGNITIVE BEHAVIOUR		
20		
21		
22		
❷❸	*	
RECEPTIVE LANGUAGE SKILLS		
24		
25		
26		
27		

ACAP – Overlay

© Helena Goldman, 2002. This form may be copied for instructional use only.

Bibliography

Aarons M & Gittens T, 1993, *The Handbook of Autism: A guide for parents and professionals*, Routledge Publications, London.

Brown W, 1994, 'The Early Years', Ellis K (ed), *Autism – Professional perspectives and practice*, Chapman & Hall, London.

Davies G, 1997, 'Communication', Powell S & Jordan R (eds), *Autism & Learning: A Guide to Good Practice*, David Fulton Publishers, London.

Dewart H and Summers S, 1988, 'The Pragmatics Profile of Early Communication Skills', NFER/Nelson, Windsor.

Fay W, 1993, 'Infantile Autism', Bishop D & Mogford K (eds), *Language Development in Exceptional Circumstances*, Laurence Erlbaum Associates Publishers, Hove.

Frith U, 1994, *Autism: Explaining the Enigma*, Blackwell Publishers, Oxford.

Goldman H, 1998, *Picture for Object Trading Communication*, unpublished paper, Birmingham.

Jordan R & Powell S, 1995, *Understanding and Teaching Children with Autism*, John Wiley & Sons Ltd, Chichester.

Jordan R, Jones G & Murray D, 1998, *Educational Interventions for Children with Autism: A Literature Review of Recent and Current Research*, Department for Education and Employment, Suffolk.

Jordan R, 1999, *An Introductory Handbook for Practitioners*, David Fulton Publishers, London.

Jordan R & Jones G, 1999, *Meeting the Needs of Children with Autistic Spectrum Disorders*, David Fulton Publishers, London.

McCall F, Markova I, Murphy J, Moodie E & Collins S, 1997, 'Perspectives on AAC systems by the users and by their communication partners', *The European Journal of Disorders of Communication* 32(3), pp235–56.

McConachie H & Pennington L, 1997, 'In-service training for schools on augmentative and alternative communication', *The European Journal of Disorders of Communication* 32(3), pp277–88.

Mesibov G, 1997, 'Formal and informal measures on the effectiveness of the TEACCH programme', *Autism: The International Journal of Research and Practice* 1(1), pp25–35.

Murphy J, Markova I, Collins S & Moodie E, 1996, 'AAC systems: obstacles to effective use', *The European Journal of Disorders of Communication* 31(1), pp31–44.

Newson E, (unpublished paper not dated) *Teaching Pointing*, 'Enabling Communication in Young Children with Autism', Early Years Diagnostic Centre, Ravenshead, Notts.

Williams D, 1996, *Autism: An Inside-Out Approach,* Jessica Kingsley Publishing Ltd, London.

Wing L, 1996, *The Autistic Spectrum: A guide for parents and professionals,* Constable & Company Ltd, London.